10 tips on herbs, spirituality and food as medicine

By Doris Richardson-Edsell, Copyright and photos by Doris Richardson-Edsell, September 12, 2014

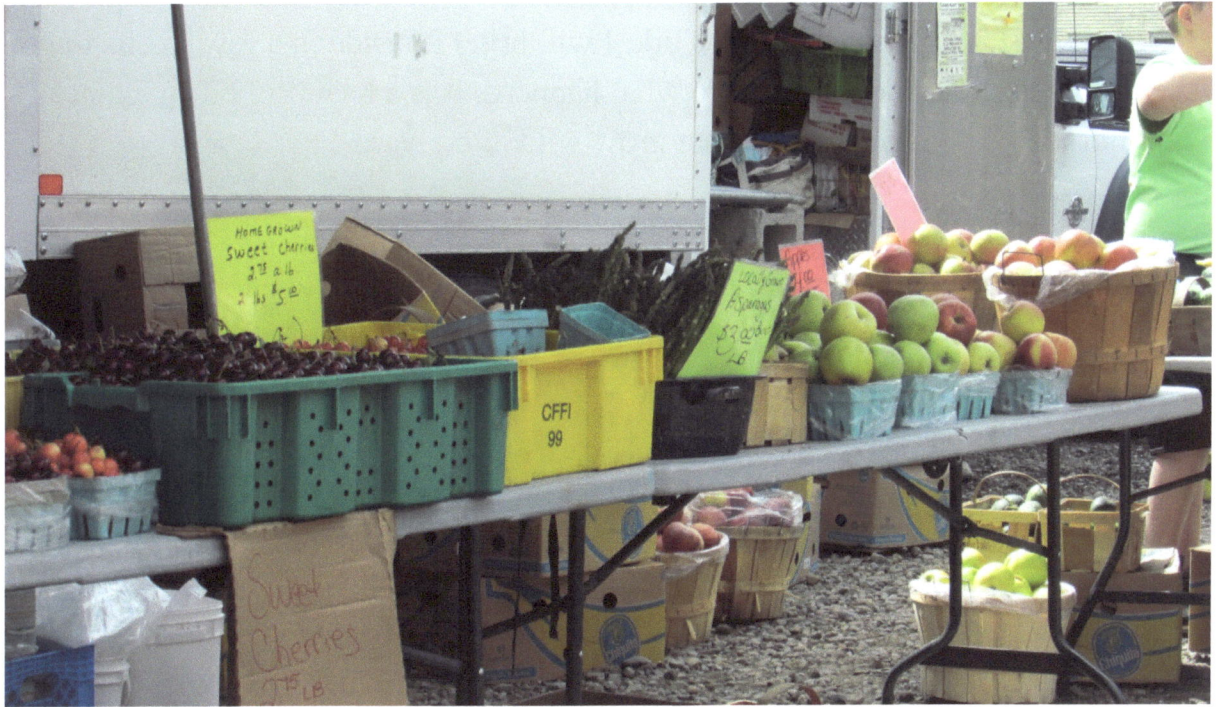

Doris Richardson-Edsell is a yoga instructor, registered nurse, writer of inspirational prose, mother and grandmother who loves to bring love, harmony and peace to the lives of others.

Staying healthy and well can include ways to use herbs and plants medicinally for some ailments in life. Just the smell of lavender helps me to stay calm and centered for the moment. Therefore it may be time for you to begin experimenting with different plants and herbs that can help you get in touch with your mind, body and soul.

Be aware that consuming live plants are similar to taking medications and other remedies; you need to know about possible side effects. Begin some self-study and look at some of the effects an herb can produce before you begin any self- help using plants and herbs. I know someone who is very allergic to lavender.

My Favorite Herbs

My personal favorite herbs are lavender, sage, thyme, basil and rosemary. They are easy to grow, especially in the summertime, and I use them in all of my recipes throughout the seasons; fresh, frozen and dried. This summer I bought my first Gogi plant because I have read about it becoming a nice berry bush for my garden, if it can live in our climate in New York. I will bring it inside in a few weeks to get it accustomed to the indoors and see what happens. It is a beautiful bushy plant with thorns like my berry bushes that grow wild in my yard.

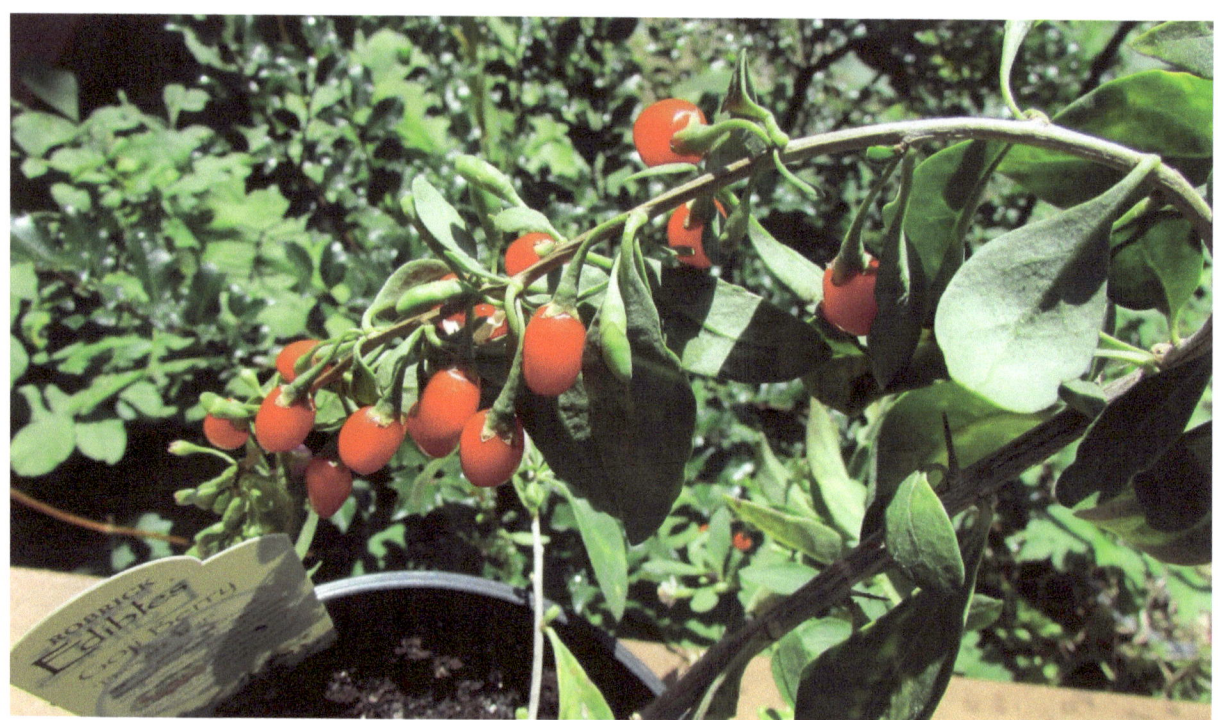

Goji Berries in my garden

1. Goji Berries

I would love to believe that Goji berries will help me to stay healthy in mind, body and soul, but the truth is that all berries are helpful antioxidants and have medicinal qualities to help you with your health and wellness.

You can also try to grow Goji berries yourself as an evergreen shrub but they are mostly found in regions that are subtropical such as China, Mongolia and in the Tibetan Himalayas. Cathy Won, ND, alternative medicine expert explains in an article: *Goji Berries: Health benefits, common uses, side effects* explains that although there are some benefits of the Goji berry such as its antioxidant effects, there are also some side effects such as not using it while taking some medicines such as blood thinners and blood pressure medicine. The Goji berry has been marketed as a helpful berry with a long history in Chinese medicine but there is currently a lack of evidence on the potential benefits of the berry but the good news is that there is some evidence including protecting the liver, helping with eyesight, improved sexual function, strengthening the legs, skin and hair health, boosting the immune system, improved circulation, promoting weight loss and promoting longevity. This is found in the author Cathy Won, ND at: http://alternativemedicine.about.com

Eyesight: Because the Goji berry is like any other berry, it is rich in antioxidant qualities particularly carotenoids such as beta-carotene and zeaxanthin. The key role in these carotenoids is to protect the eyes, as do eating carrots but many healthy Goji tonics have been created which are expensive and may be unnecessary in helping with your health and wellness. The only test on humans appears to be in a Chinese study in 1994, published in the Chinese Journal of Oncology. They found that 79 people responded better to cancer treatments when Goji was added to their regimen. There needs to be more research on the topic of the use of Goji berries however there also have been some test tube studies which have been promising on using Goji berry extract to stop the growth of cancer cells, reduce blood glucose levels and cholesterol levels but this does not mean that humans will have the same benefit if taken as a juice or tea.

2. Quiet

Every once in a while I listen to the silence of things. That is why I grow herbs. They silently help me, and along the way I get to enjoy their potent smells and medicinal ways. Just the smell of fresh herbs in the garden can be a mood enhancer.

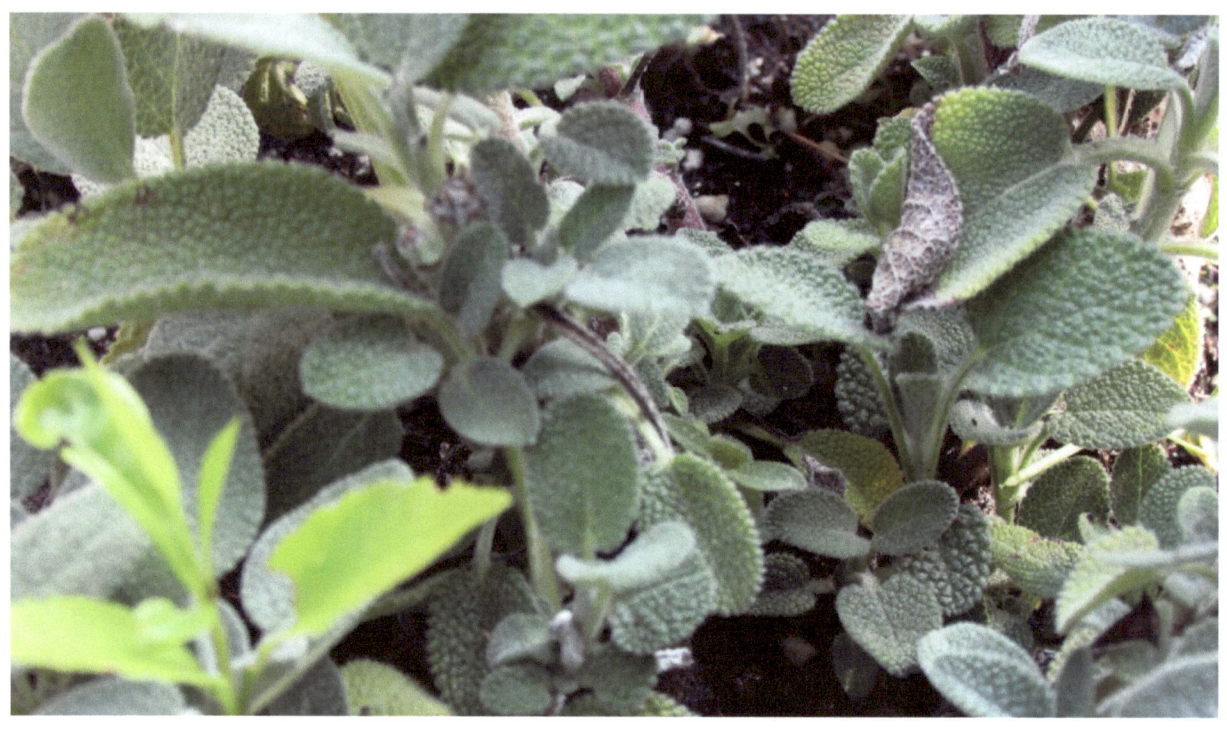

Sage helps with so many ailments- even the night sweats of menopause

When I was younger I felt like I never had silence in my life. I always had children around me, making noise and chattering! I loved to hear their tiny voices and still enjoy it when I am with my grandchildren. The difference now is that I also enjoy the silence. Not having to speak early in the day is one of my favorite times. And in the summertime I can sit on my back porch and just be; watching my herbs and greeting the sunny days. One of my favorites is Sage and today I decided to study it. I just love the smell, and I mix it up for an easy salad dressing with olive oil and my other herbs. I also use it as a pesto on my noodle dishes in the summertime.

Easy Sage, Basil and Thyme Recipe

In a food processor or blender place a handful of your favorite herbs. Today I used Sage, Basil and Thyme (about 4 leaves of each basil and sage, and a small branch of thyme.) I blended them with 1/2 cup water and 2 teaspoons of lemon juice; after blended I added 1/4 cup Extra Virgin olive oil, blended again, and then added a chopped clove of garlic. It was wonderful on my lunch salad. And what I saved for later will be even better because for some reason after it settles in the refrigerator, it thickens up a bit.

Some sage tips:

1. Sage tea for fever and to relieve nervous tension

2. Sage juice in warm water for hoarseness and coughs

Herbalist also use sage to treat sprains, swelling, ulcers and bleeding

3. The Chinese valued sage for the stomach and nervous system including weakness of digestion in general. Beneficial in liver complaints, kidney troubles, colds in the head as well as sore throat, pain in the joints. It is well documented that sage can help with menopausal sweats.

It is thought that Sage is similar to Rosemary in its ability to improve brain function and memory. In a study involving 20 healthy volunteers, Sage oil caused indicated improvements in word recall and speed of attention, and there is continuing investigation with sage in the search for new drugs to help with Alzheimer's disease. Wouldn't it be wonderful if an herb like Sage could stop the progression of Alzheimer's disease?

From www.herbwisdom.com/herb-sage.html:

3. Insomnia

You may know that insomnia can be directly related to how much stress you have in your life, so the first thing to do is try to decrease it. This may take some time, and exercise of any type is very helpful. I suggest the passive ones for insomniacs because you learn about slowing everything down and you can do the poses of tai chi or yoga anytime and anywhere. Settle down in the evening with a lavender eye pillow over your eyes, lying down before you go to bed. I sometimes take lavender pillows with me to bed for the comforting effects.

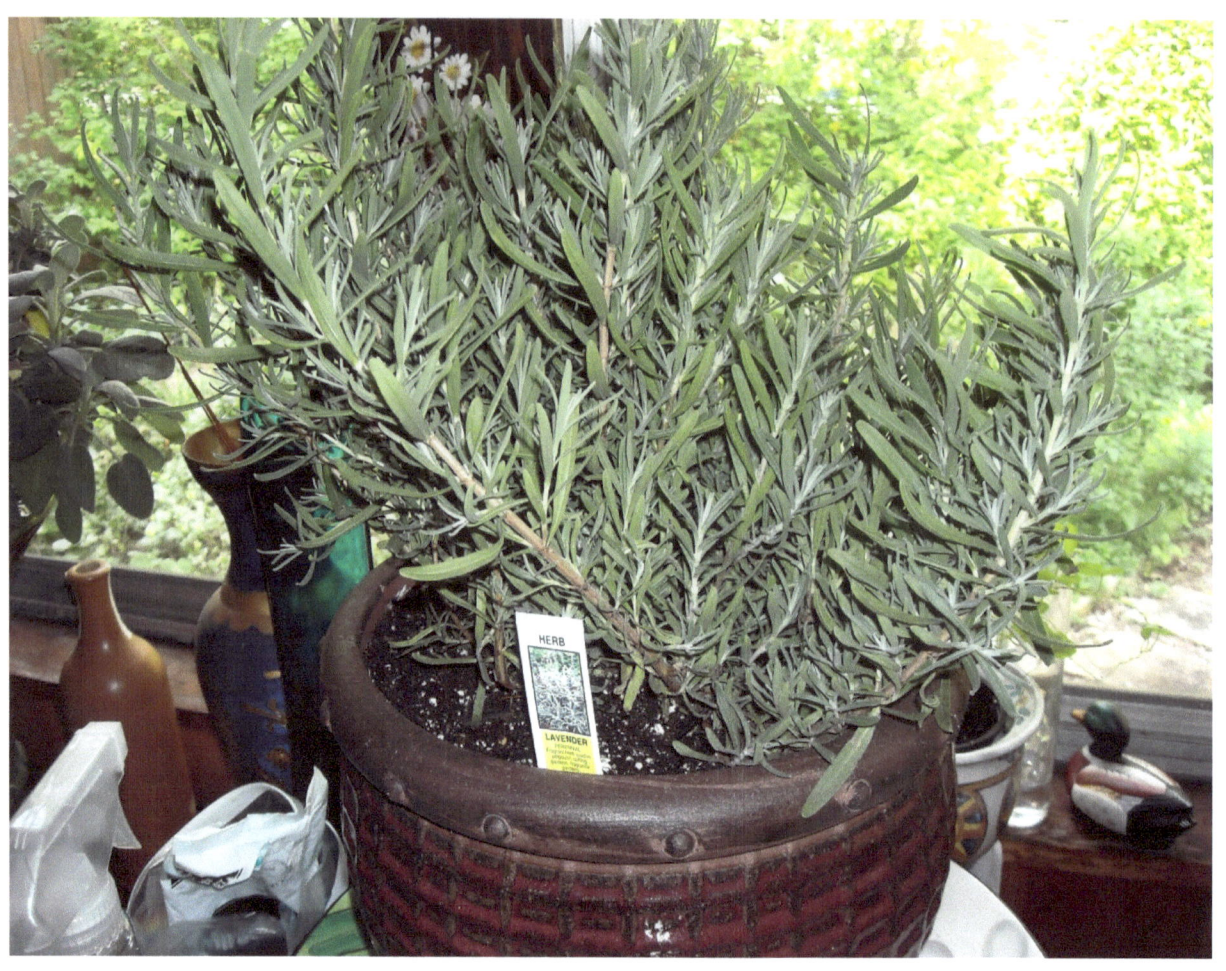

Lavender, such a soothing herb for the skin

In a booklet on aromatherapy entitled: Aromatherapy: *It's Not an Old Wives' Tale Anymore;* Bernie Ward describes how oils such as lavender can help with sleep. Oils that are calming include lavender, Roman chamomile, sandalwood, juniper berry and ylang-ylang.

All you need is a few drops in your bath or a tiny drop behind your neck before bed. I use lavender because it is so soothing to the skin.

You can also blend all of these oils together. ***Here is a recipe:***

3 drops lavender, 3 drops ylang-ylang, 2 drops Roman Chamomile and 2.5 teaspoons of carrier oil.

Before going to bed, massage your face, neck and shoulders with this mixture! Lavender is a great plant to grow. It is powerful in many ways: treating burns, a natural antibiotic and detoxifier. Lavender can stimulate the immune system. As an antidepressant and sleep inducer, lavender can help with insomnia. Taken in part from: Ward, B. (1995) Aromatherapy: *It's Not an Old Wives' Tale Anymore.* Boca, Raton, Fl. Globe Communications

4. Why you should use Garlic

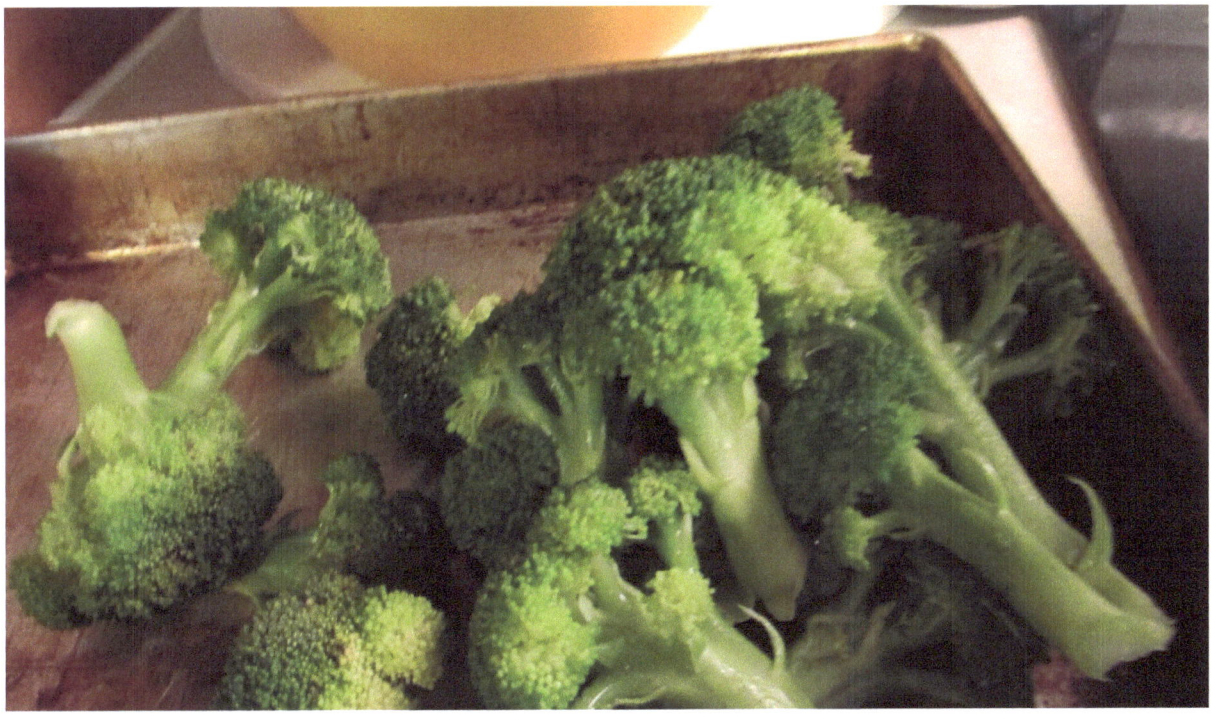

Add some fresh ginger and garlic to your broccoli before roasting

In the winter I have time to experiment with some spices. I enjoy both garlic and ginger together in many of my meals. Try adding some fresh garlic to your dishes.

GARLIC

A phytonutrient and a star spice

Garlic can improve cardiovascular health; lower the risk of cancer, and help fight infection. Garlic can even improve the safety of your barbecue. A great tip about garlic for your summer grilling:
You can improve the safety of your meat dishes that you cook on the grill by cooking them with garlic. When high protein foods are cooked on a barbecue, they release a chemical known as Ph1P, a toxic substance that is linked to cancer.
A study done with women who eat large amounts of barbecued meats had a significant increase in cancer. When a phytonutrient called diallylsufide DAS, one of the sulfide compounds that gives garlic its characteristic smell, can inhibit the carcinogenic effects of Ph1P. DAS protects DNA from damage and stops the conversion of Ph1P in the body into other carcinogenic substances. When

researchers in Florida A&M University in Tallahassee treated breast cells of rats with Ph1P, and then added DAS, the garlic compound stopped the cancer process. Taken in part from: Watson, B. (2007) *The Fiber 35 Diet: Nature's Weight Loss Secret.* New York, NY. Free Press.

5. Remedies that help skin problems

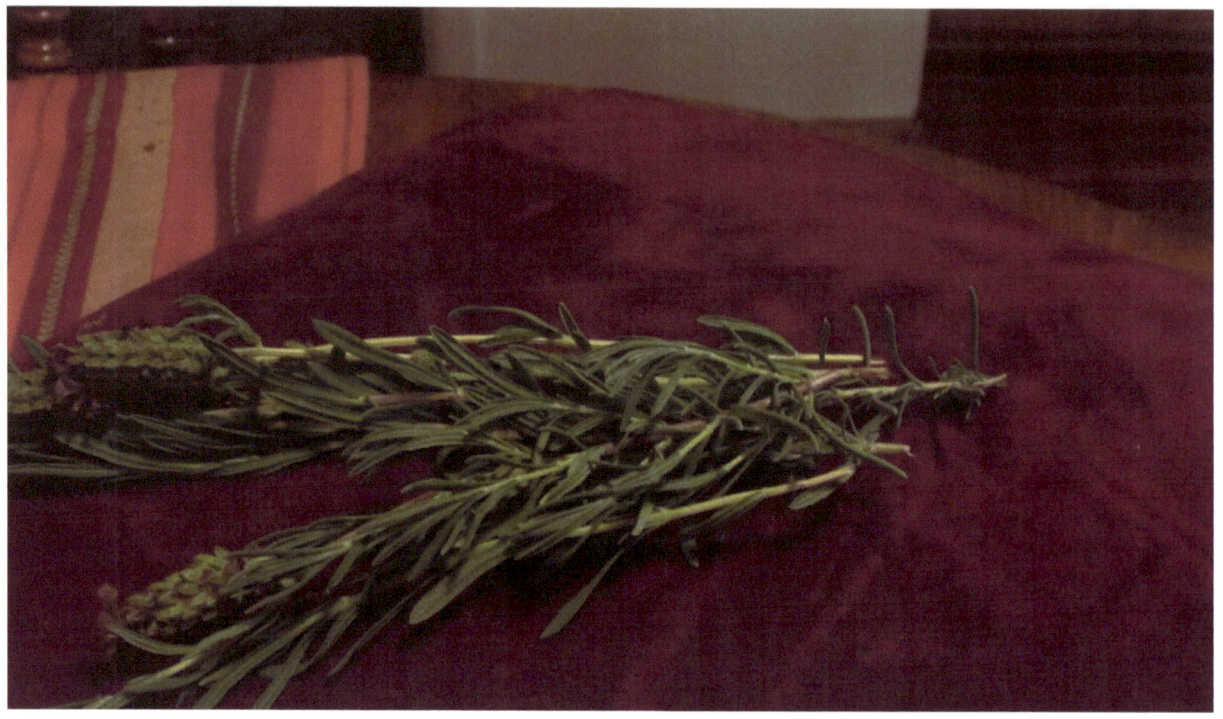

Weeds and herbs can be wonderful for helping your skin. French Lavender is softer and smoother to the touch.

Here are some remedies for some minor skin problems.

Starting with ACNE: Some first steps to help

Most of the time acne is from too much sebum (oil) on the skin. This oil can bring about bacteria, causing plugged hair follicles in skin pores.

If it lodges near the surface of the skin, blackheads and whiteheads will form. If a blockage ruptures, it becomes a pimple.

Sometimes the problem is hormonal, stress, diet or irritating ingredients in makeup.

What to do?

Acne, pimples and spots: Reach for the weeds first:

1. Yarrow is a true remedy for acne. For a yarrow infusion, placed dried yarrow flowers into a quart jar and fill with boiling water. Steep overnight, strain and store in a plastic bottle. Dampen a washcloth with it every morning, evening and in between!

2. Burdock seed or root

An Herbalist, Susan Weed believes that brewing up some burdock can help. You can use it to clean the skin. " For acne rosacea, take 10-20 drops of burdock seed or root tincture three times a day, which will bring slow but steady improvement." You can buy burdock tincture at a health food store. It is called Actium Lappa. You can also make it into a very strong tea from dried burdock root, brew overnight and drink a few cups a day.

3. Take an herbal steam bath

Herbal steaming opens embedded pores. You can use a combination of herbs such as yarrow, elder flowers and chamomile. Put these herbs into a large pot, cover with a quart of cool water and bring to a slow simmer. Cover the pot with a towel and your head so that the steam touches your face, keeping your eyes closed. Remember not to get too close, you do not want to burn yourself. Steam for about 15 minutes.

Natural First Aid for Burns bruises, cuts and scrapes

Here are some remedies that work for burns and minor cuts

The aloe Vera plant: For soothing a minor burn, including sunburn, try some aloe. You can use some fresh aloe by snapping off a piece from a mature plant and applying the transparent gel to your skin. Aloe has also been used as a first aid for frost bite because it acts against thromboxanes, a substance that constricts blood vessels. When aloe is applied, the blood vessels relax, helping to heal the frost bite.

Lavender: This plant can help with minor cuts and scrapes. Mix 15 drops of lavender essential oil with an ounce of Aloe Vera juice. They are both available at a health food store. Place the mixture in a spray bottle and store in the refrigerator for a soothing, cool mist that you can spray on minor cuts and scrapes.

Promoting healing with Plantain: This common weed can be found in most lawns and it can help to soothe pain, bind together torn tissue and strengthen the skin's surface. When used fresh, crush a few thin leaves and apply to minor cuts and scrapes. At the health food store, you can also find some plantain salve to ease itching and promote healing.

Taken in part from: Fugh-Berman, A. (1998). *Women's Choices in Natural Healing. Drug-Free Remedies from the World of Alternative Medicine.* Emmaus, PA. Rodale Press, Inc.

Taken in part from: Haas, E. (2003) Staying healthy with the Seasons. 21st Century Edition. San Rafeal, CA. Random House.

6. Summer Spices and herbs

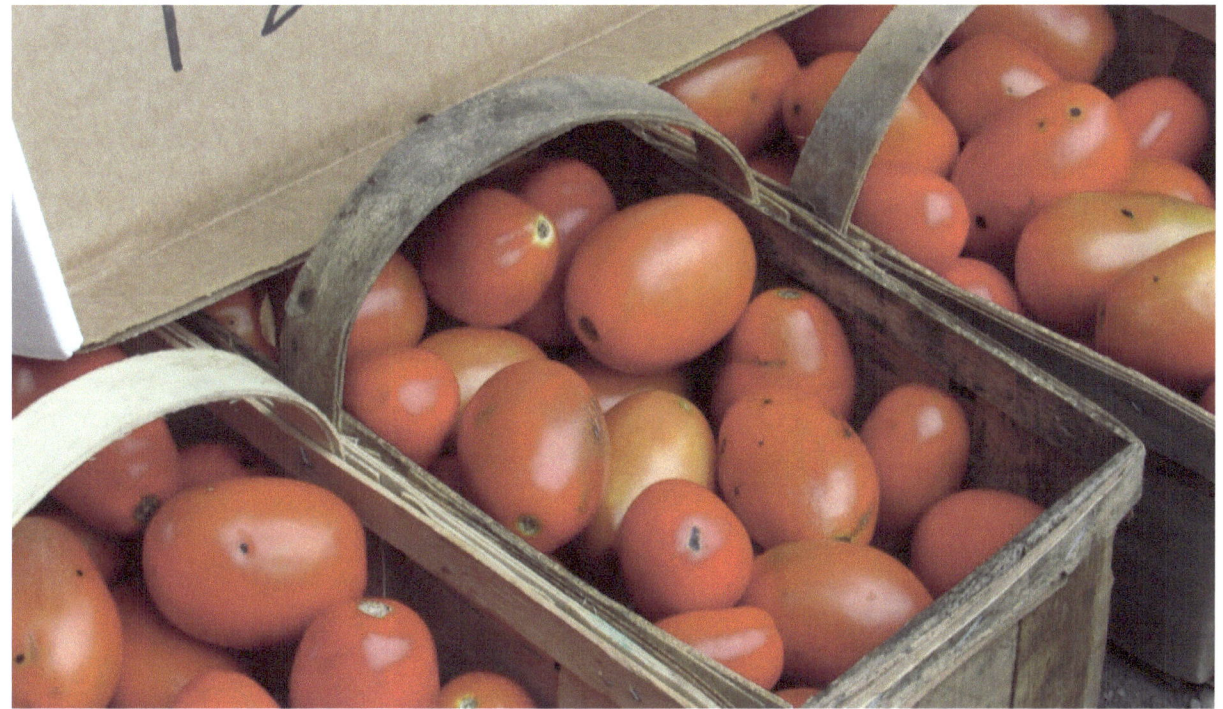

Making your own salsa can be fun with some spices such as cayenne pepper to spice up a simple salsa

Chop some ripe tomatoes, about 2 cups and then add your spices such as cumin and cayenne pepper. Then chop a clove of garlic and 1 white onion. Allow your salsa to sit in the refrigerator overnight and you will have a great salsa. Summertime is the time to strengthen your Fire Element. Taking in some sun will help, along with exercise, healthy foods and some good herbs!

Cayenne pepper is one of nature's true stimulants. Medicinally, it is known as a tonic of sorts. It provides us with energy and acts as a heating agent, without being irritating. It makes a good healer for wounds and sores and for an irritated or ulcerated stomach or colon. Cayenne pepper is a good herb for colds, flu, and sore throats, plus helpful in weak circulation. Cayenne pepper is a heart stimulant which acts as a blood cleanser, and may aid in the elimination of impurities from the blood by increasing the urine flow and by sweating. It has also been used to treat problems of the kidneys, spleen and pancreas.

Ginger Root, another common herb that is very aromatic. Ginger root has been used for suppressed menstruation, colds, sore throats, diarrhea, indigestion and nausea.

Hot greens like mustard, watercress, cauliflower or cabbage stimulate the Fire; while garlic is good for strong, clean blood.

Try some cooling fruit juices like orange or lemonade or try some cooling herbs such as mint and many of the flowers such as hibiscus and chamomile flowers. Boil some water and pour into a pot with one of several of these herbs and let steep for 20-30 minutes.

Solar teas

All of the herbs can also be made into *solar teas* by placing some herbs into a glass jug with water and leaving it out in the sunlight for a day. Examples of which herbs to use: peppermint, Hibiscus flower, Lemongrass, Red Clover Flowers, Chamomile Flowers, Rosemary, Orange or lemon peel.

Fire Element and hot foods from Haas, E. (2003) *Staying Healthy With the Seasons.* Celestial Arts, San Rafael, CA.

7. In the autumn of your Life

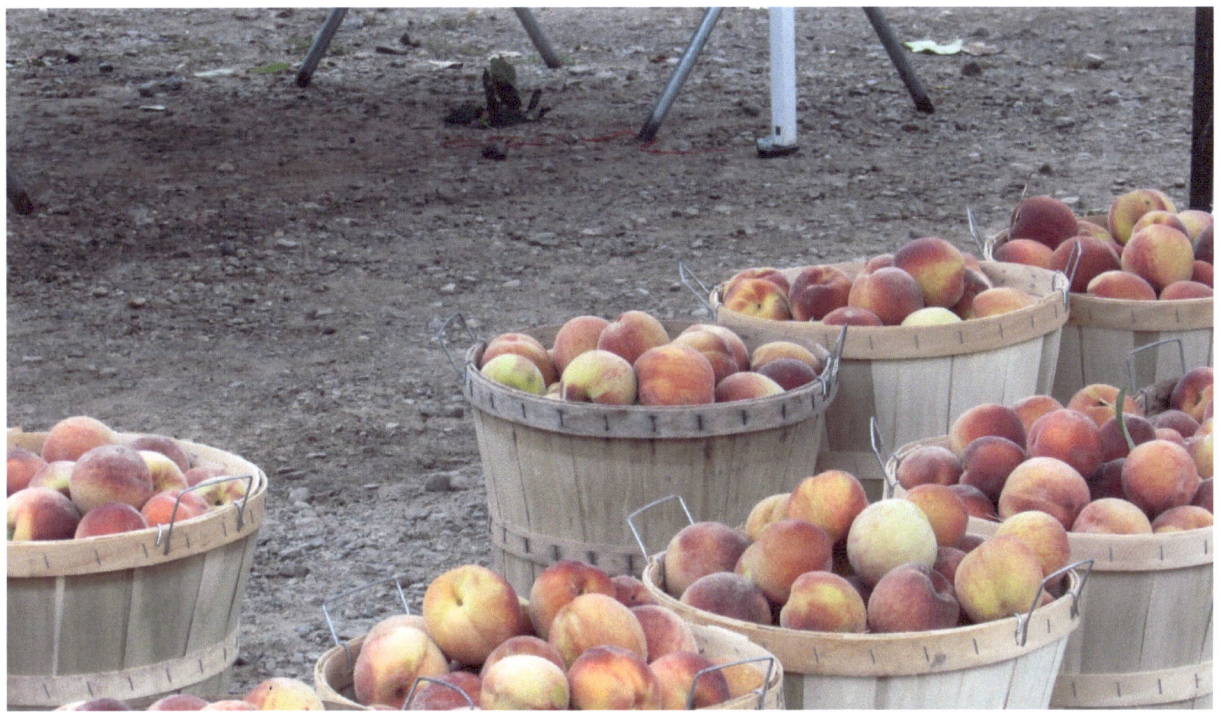

At the end of the season it is time for canning and preserving for winter months

What should we be eating?

Think about what you are eating, and how much while you head toward the fall and winter. We have to cut down this time of year, and just the thought of cutting back may be difficult. I have found that the bright, golden and orange veggies in my diet this time of year is helpful, because they are filling. For example, a steamed or baked sweet potato adds to my lunch, while some acorn squash with cinnamon and a little stevia can make my steamed squash taste great. Autumn should also be a cleansing time of year when we get rid of things, pack things away and change our clothing to more suitable sweaters for the cool evenings if we live on the east coast. The crisp time of year is the time for soups, exercise and herbs.

Here are a few Herbs that are helpful in the autumn

Here are a few herbs that can energize you in the fall. As we start to feel less active we need to turn to the root herbs.

Burdock root as a tonic is helpful for the skin.

Comfrey- is both root and leaf, but is known as one of the great healing plants. High in protein, vitamins and minerals, it can be used for healing and cleansing wounds. The fresh leaf can be used for wrap on sprains. The comfrey root can be taken daily as a tea.

Ginger-For some body heat, try some ginger root, sliced and simmered for 15-20 minutes, and then mix with other herbs. Ginger can also help with circulation and cold areas on the body. Just apply a cloth or towel, soaked in warm ginger root tea.

Cayenne pepper- Putting some cayenne pepper in your diet in the fall can keep you warm. Some people put it in their socks to help warm their feet.

Herb news, taken in part from: Haas, E. (2003) *Staying Healthy with the Seasons.* 21st Ed. San Rafael, CA. Celestial Arts.

8. *Autumn Foods*

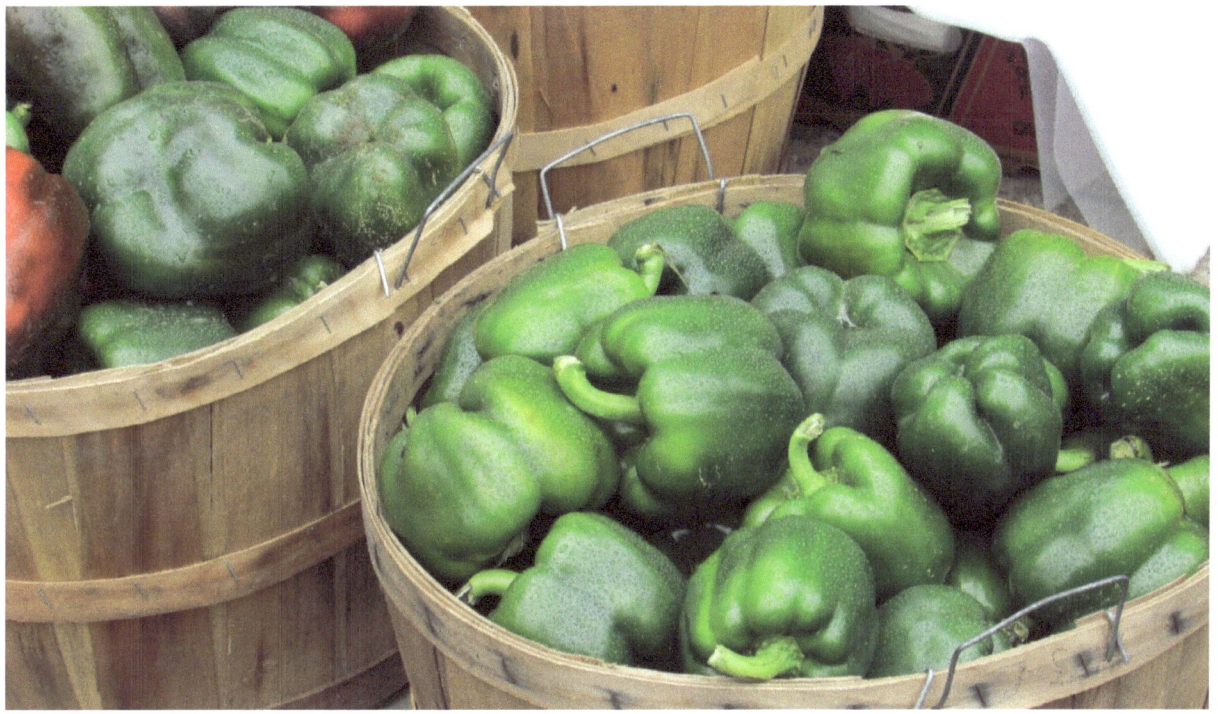

Green peppers, so delicious in the fall

There are so very many autumn foods, and they are colorful and good for you. Try out some new squashes. I have found that many of them are different. Even the different colors for sweet peppers are amazing. I just bought some purple peppers!

What a better way to experiment with the great autumn harvest. I bought some large apples at the farmer's market this week, and the person selling them said they were great for baking. But I just bite right into one, and thought it was great!

Dr.Elson Haas in his book, *Staying Healthy with the Seasons* believes that seasonal changes should bring about changes in what we eat.

For some balance in your diet in the fall season: Builders: beans and animal proteins, Cleansers include fruits and vegetables. Sweets, cheese and breads; you need small amounts, especially nuts, seeds and oils.

Some suggestions for what to eat

Bake some squash or pumpkin and stuff it with a combination of already cooked brown and wild rice along with some almonds and mushrooms. This is simple, and a great autumn dish. In the crisp autumn weather, some soup may be another easy suggestion.

Soup

Add some vegetables such as carrots, turnip, onions, and garlic to some soaking barley. Follow directions on the barley packaging for cooking times, rinsing and draining.

At the end of the cooking time, add some greens such as kale, celery and spinach. Then allow simmering. Sea veggies such as dulse, kelp, or nori seaweed as well as miso paste can give the broth some flavor.

Creamy soups: Make some pumpkin or squash soup. Just steam some squash, mash it adding some milk or almond milk, which I prefer. Add some spices such as rosemary, cayenne, ginger or your own favorites.

9. *Toward winter months: Time to keep yourself healthy and well*

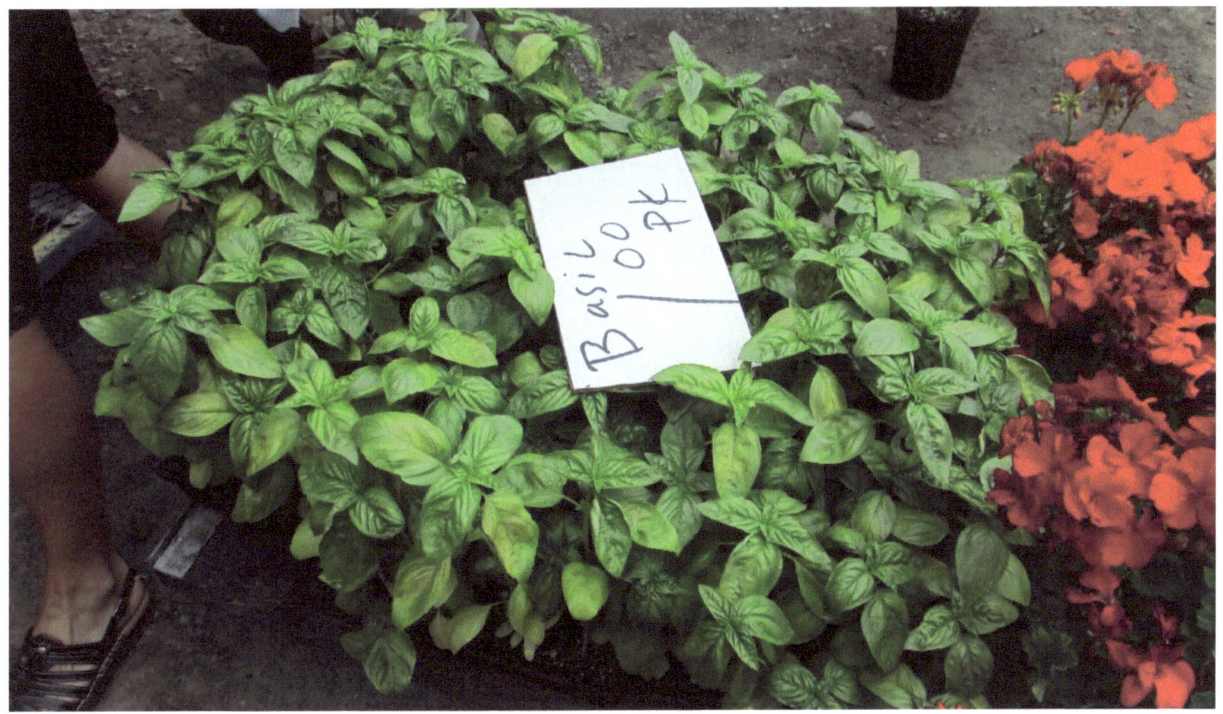

Get some basil at your local farmer's market; freeze it or dry it and use it all winter

Take some long walks during autumn to see the wonderful colors. And eat some colorful foods such as squash and sweet potatoes. They keep you healthy and well!

Keeping those extra pounds away for the winter months

This is the time of year when people begin to put on the pounds, so care needs to be taken in what you eat. There are very nutritious foods for the fall and winter months that can not only keep you healthy and well, but can also help with weight maintenance.

Weight Maintenance: Make some soup

Staying the same weight in the winter as you were in the summer can be difficult. I try to stick with soups. They seem to satisfy me more in the winter, plus keep me warm. It has been written by many authors that people who eat soup are thinner than people who don't. So plan on some different recipes, and experiment with the veggies that you love.

Creamy soups

You do not have to use cream or whole milk to make creamy and delicious, low calorie soup.

I use milk alternatives such as almond milk to make my soups creamier. I usually put them in as the last ingredient after the soup has simmered. For example, sweet potato soup can be chunky or creamy, depending on what you do with it. I like it both ways, and a combination. I cook some sweet potatoes until tender, and allow cooling. Mash or cream them in a blender. Simmer for about 10 minutes. Then stir in some almond milk. This type of soup can be served hot or cold.

Veggie Soup

I start my veggie soups with a can of V8 juice (low sodium)

I use the small cans. The 4 ounce can with another 4 ounces of water make a great start to a healthy veggie soup. I begin by adding the vegetables that take longer to cook such as fresh carrots. Whatever your pleasure, the more veggies, the better. For a heartier soup, I add quinoa, my favorite grain. You can also add some pasta instead.

Salads

Give your salads some extra ingredients in the cooler months

For my lettuce salads in the winter, I do not use tomatoes because they do not taste that great in the winter, and I add black olives, artichoke hearts and some chick peas. For my winter dressings I use oil and vinegar (half and half) with a touch of fresh ginger chopped finely. I also make some citrus dressings made out of tangerines and/or grapefruit juice with a pinch of fresh garlic, sage and basil.

De-Stressing Methods in the Winter Months

To keep yourself stress free in the winter months, you can also try some aromatherapy for you baths, or for spraying around the house. Since we are indoors more in the winter months, experimenting with some essential oils can be helpful to your health. Here are a few tips from the book: *Women's Choices in Natural Healing* by author Adriane Fugh-Burgman.

Basil- nature's nerve tonic. Mix 5 drops of pure essential basil oil into a thimbleful of alcohol with 4 ounces of distilled water and place in a clear spray bottle. Store in the refrigerator. Shake well before using and avoid your eyes.

Clary sage- the mood elevator. Clary sage oil is a great mood elevator, but do not mix with alcohol.

Geranium – hormonal balancer. When added to your bath or mixed in your lotion. It can balance mood swings and ease depression.

Oil references taken from: Fugh-Berman, A. (1998) *Women's Choices in Natural Healing.* Emmaus, PA. Rodale Press.

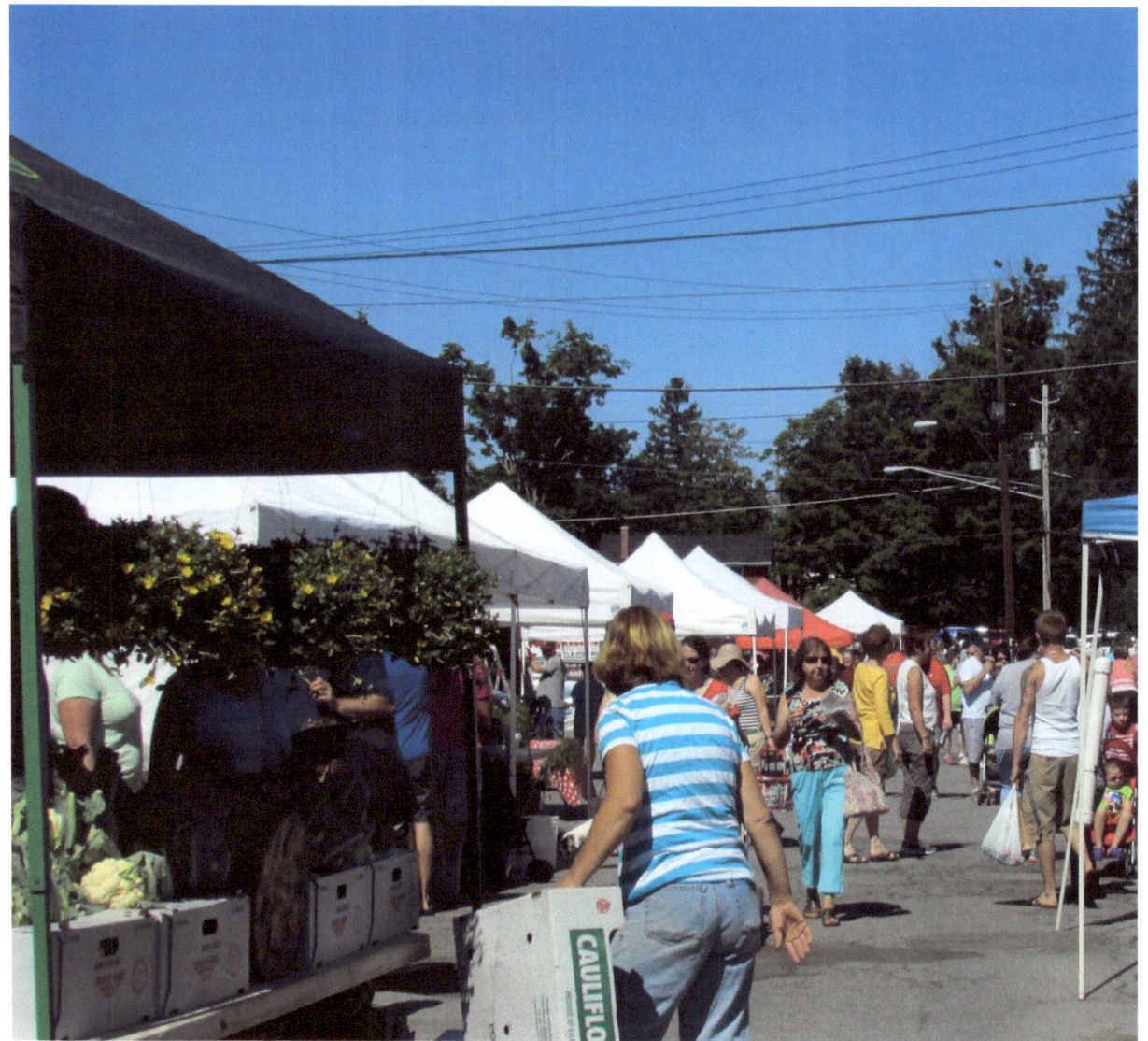

Healing through your spirit

10. Spiritual Growth in your life

Sometimes your spirit needs to grow through touching nature and taking care of living things that grow. Walking through a Farmer's Market in the fall will bring your spirit out to see the wonders of eating fresh and healthy. There is much evidence on the positive effects of spirituality and meditation as a healing way to get in touch with your inner soul, bringing lasting peace and harmony into your life.

Your spirit rises to see the blue sky from above looking down at the world, and there is a moment when you can see your shadow and how it helps you in life. That spiritual body is there for you; bringing you comfort in sad times and laughter in happy times. There is so much more than living life physically, and you will find this to be more and more apparent as you age. As time passes, your spiritual sense of life becomes the stronger piece of your many *selves*, telling you it is time to find your place in life and in death. And if death scares you right now, it will not be that way when you move closer to death; not welcoming it, but accepting the abundance of your life and the wonders of your next life as a spirit.

Meditate

Take yourself away on your spiritual path through some meditative practices that calm the mind, body and soul. Staying healthy includes finding healing ways through the many alternative modalities; beginning with meditation and prayer.

Do not rush yourself with learning some new ways. Meditation and relaxation techniques take time to learn just like any other skill you can focus on; practice and you will get better; finding peaceful moments instead of stressful times. It has been well researched that the largest cause of inflammation and general sickness in the body is from psychological stress, so you need to do some things that helps you.

Breathe

Learning how to slow yourself down through some breathing exercises is important to your health and wellness throughout your life. Deep, slow, breathing in through the nose for the count of 5 and out through the mouth for the count of 7 with an *ah (open mouth)* sound can get you on the way to more effective breathing; slowing you breath, your blood pressure and your mind. When you begin your breathing practice, you slow yourself down and become more mindful of your being; concentrating on you, the person who needs to take care of their mind, body and spirit.

What is your spiritual being?

Finding ways to be one with your internal self can be a life- long event where you learn how your spirit is connected to your mind and body. Living a more spiritual life can be a good goal for anyone. When you combine learning about nature, growing your own herbs, vegetables and fruits, you realize how important all living things are. When you learn how to nurture plants, you will know how to be more nurturing and loving to others in your life path. Kindness, love and caring for yourself and others becomes a natural exploration that you embrace every day of your life.

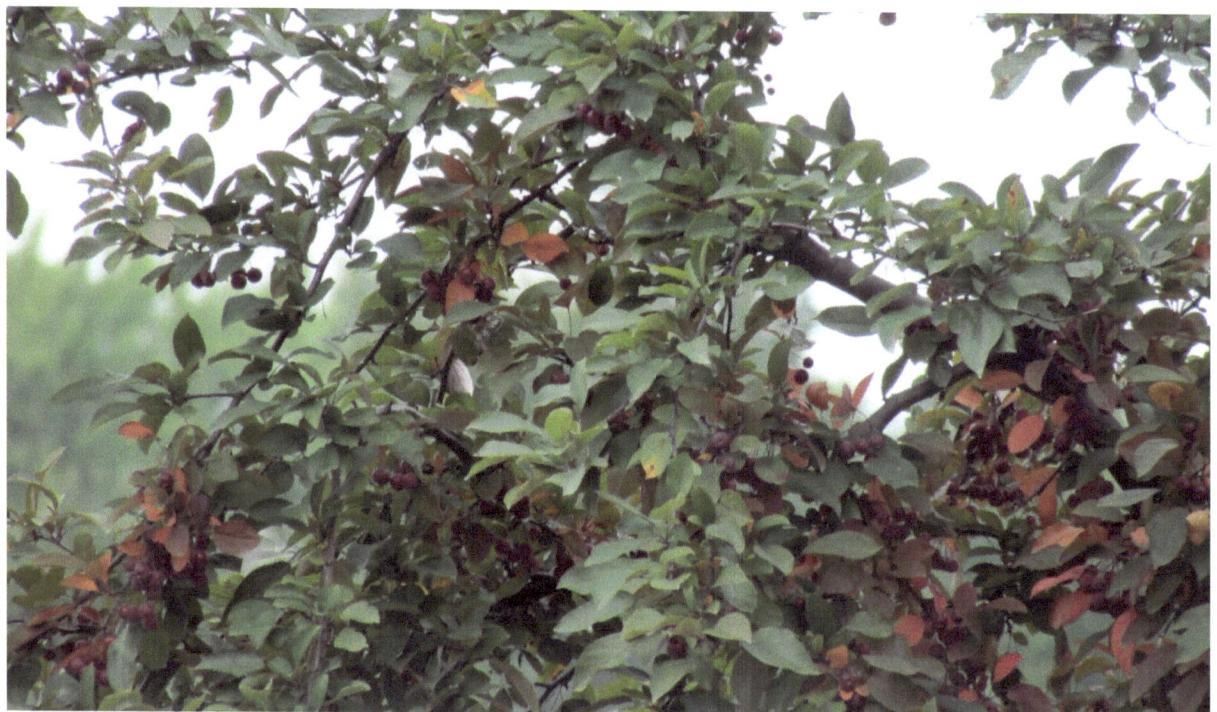

Trees tell the story of life and living because they are strong and flexible, the way we would like to be

A new dimension to your life

Learning about yourself and beginning self-care techniques can be a new dimension to your life where you begin to realize how important it is to just be; not caught up the stressful events of life which can limit your happiness and joy. Because what else is there in life besides being happy?

Making sense of life and death

Death seems a lot like birth, but just the opposite dimension. That is probably why there is a saying, "when one person dies, another is born."

I believe that there is no way to prepare for the many changes in life and approaching the later years can be difficult especially if you are struggling with illness. Hopefully decline will be slow for you because you take good care of yourself.

And whatever it is that brings you to your last breath, remember the significance of life and how you are spending your time in the here and now of living life well.

Your life expectations

If you help others, your life will change because life is like a circle filled with energy. And when your positive energy goes around it comes back to you in so many different loving ways.

What good can you do right now?

Doris

Bibliography

For more information on herbs, plants and their many uses:

Fiber- Watson, B. (2007). The Fiber 35 Diet: Nature's Weight loss Secret. New York, NY. Free Press.

Goji- http://alternativemedicine.about.com

Herb news, taken in part from: Haas, E. (2003) *Staying Healthy with the Seasons.* 21st Ed. San Rafael, CA. Celestial Arts.

Oil references taken from: Fugh-Berman, A. (1998) *Women's Choices in Natural Healing.* Emmaus, PA. Rodale Press.

Sage- www.herbwisdom.com

Ward, B. (1995). *Aromatherapy*: *It's Not an Old Wives' Tale Anymore*. Boca, Raton, Fl. Globe Communications.